1

LUNG CANCER

All about Lung Cancer, Types, Medical prescriptions and possible cure: Also guide for caregivers, patients, & health professionals

DR. KATE D. MARTINS

(Ph.D.)

PREFACE

If you enjoy this book, please try to leave a review.

Also send me your thoughts and considerations about this book. That includes what you think is missing or what needs to be added in this book through this mail: ws905360@gmail.com and you will get a FREE copy of my next book.

Table of Content

INTRODUCTION

THE HISTORY OF LUNG CANCER

Lung cancer was unusual before the advent of cigarette smoking. Great surgeon Alton Ochsner recalled that as a Washington University medical student in 1919, his entire medical school class was called to witness an examination (autopsy) of a man who had died from cancer of the lungs, and told that they may never see such a case again. In Adler's 1912 Primary Malignant Growths of the Lungs and Bronchi, he called lung cancer "among the uncommon and rare forms of disease"; Adler also tabulated all the 374 cases of lung cancer that had been published to that time, concluding the disease was increasing in occurrences. In the late 1920s, several theories had been brought forth, connecting the increase in lung cancer to various chemical exposures and pollution that had increased including industrial air pollution, tobacco smoke, asphalt dust, and poisonous gasses from World War I.

Throughout the following years, developing scientific proof connected lung cancer to cigarette consumption. In the 1940s and mid-1950s, a few case-control studies showed that those with cellular breakdown in the lungs (lung cancer) were more likely to have smoked cigarettes compared with those without lung cancer. These were connected by a few cohort studies during the 1950s - including the initial report of the British Specialists in 1954 - all of which proved that the people who smoked tobacco were at high risk of developing lung cancer.

A report from the year 1953 (which showed that tar from tobacco smoke could cause cancers in mice) stood out and attracted attention in the famous press, which featured in life and Time magazines.

Confronting public concern and falling stock costs, the Chiefs of six of the biggest American tobacco organizations had a meeting in December 1953. They enrolled the assistance of public relation firm, Hill and Knowlton to create a multi-pronged strategies whose sole purpose is to divert and distract from gathering proof by financing tobacco-accommodating examination and research, proclaiming the connection to lung cancer "dubious/controversial", and requesting more research to settle this implied controversy. Simultaneously, internal exploration and research at the major tobacco organizations backed the connection between tobacco and lung cancer; however these outcomes or results were hidden from the public.

As proof connecting tobacco use with lung cancer increased, different health bodies and organizations reported official positions connecting the two. In the year 1962, Royal College of Physicians, United Kingdom authoritatively reached a conclusion that cigarette smoking causes lungs cancer, causing the US Top health Surgeon general to empanel (select or enlist) a warning and advisory committee, which thought covertly over 9 meetings between November 1962 and December 1963. The committee report, distributed in January 1964, immovably presumed that cigarette smoking passes by far any other variables and factors in causing lung cancer. The report got coverage in the press, and is broadly viewed as a defining moment for public acknowledgment that tobacco smoking causes lung cancer.

The link with radon gas was first perceived in excavators in Germany's Mineral Mountains. Miners were observed to develop a destructive illness called "mountain disorder" (Bergkrankheit), identified as lung cancer by the late nineteenth century. By 1938, up to 80% of miners in areas that were already affected died from the disease. In the early 1950s, radon and its breakdown items became laid out as reasons for cellular breakdown in the lungs (lung cancer) in miners. Dependent generally upon studies of miners, the International Agency for Research on Cancer classified radon as "carcinogenic" to people in 1988. In 1956, a review revealed radon in Swedish homes. Throughout the next few years, high radon concentrations were tracked down in homes across the world; by the 1980s numerous nations had laid out public radon projects to list and relieve private radon.

The first fruitful and successful pneumonectomy for lung cancer, in 1933 by Evarts Graham at Barnes Hospital in St. Louis, Missouri. Throughout the following years, surgical improvement zeroed in on saving however much healthy lung tissue as possible, with the lobectomy outperforming the pneumonectomy in recurrence by the 1960s, and the wedge resection showing up in the mid 1970s. This pattern went on with the advancement of video-assisted thoracoscopic surgical procedures in the 1980s, presently generally performed for some cellular breakdown in the lung surgeries.

CHAPTER 1
SIGNS & SYMPTOMS

Usually, early lung cancer has no signs and symptoms. At the point when symptoms really do emerge they are in many cases vague respiratory issues - chest pain, coughing, and shortness of breath - that can vary from individual to person. The people who experience coughing will usually report either another cough, or a high level recurrence or strength of a prior cough. Around one of every four cough up blood, going from little streaks in the sputum to larger amounts. Around half of those diagnosed to have lung cancer experience shortness of breath, while from 30-50% tend to experience a dull, aggressive chest pain that reoccur in the same area over time. Notwithstanding respiratory symptom, some experience systemic symptom including:

- *Weight loss,*
- *Weakness,*
- *Loss of appetite,*

☐ *Fever, and*

☐ *Night sweats.*

A few more unusual symptoms tend to suggest cancer specific areas. Growths in the thorax can cause breathing issues by impeding the trachea or disturbing the nerve to the diaphragm (stomach); trouble in swallowing by compressing the throat; roughness by upsetting the nerves of the larynx; and Horner's condition by disturbing the sympathetic nervous system. Horner's disorder is likewise normal in growths at the top point of the lung, known as Pancoast cancers, which likewise cause shoulder pain that emanates down the little-finger, side of the arm, as well as obliteration of the highest ribs. Swollen lymph nodes over the collarbone indicates a growth that has spread inside the chest. Growths disrupting blood flow to the heart can cause predominant vena cava disorder (shortness of breath and swelling of the chest area), while cancers penetrating the region around the heart can cause fluid development and build up around the heart, arrhythmia (sporadic heartbeat), and heart failure.

Around 1 out of 3 individuals diagnosed to have lung cancer have signs and symptoms brought about by metastases in parts other than the lungs. Lung cancer can metastasize anywhere in the body, with various signs and symptoms depending on the area. Cerebrum (brain) metastases can cause seizures, nausea, headache, vomiting, and neurological shortages. Bone metastases can cause pain, bone fracture, and pressure of the spinal cord. Metastasis into the bone marrow can deplete platelets (blood cells) and cause leukoerythroblastosis (juvenile cells in the blood). Liver metastases can cause liver expansion, pain in the right upper quadrant of the abdomen, fever, and weight loss.

Lung growths frequently cause the release of body-altering hormones, which cause uncommon signs and symptoms, called paraneoplastic syndromes. Unseemly hormone release can cause dramatic changes in groupings of blood minerals. Most usual is hypercalcemia (high blood calcium) brought about by overproduction of parathyroid or hormone related protein. . Hypercalcemia can manifest as vomiting, nausea, abdominal pain, constipation, increased thirst, frequent urination, and altered mental status. Those with cellular breakdown in the lungs likewise generally experience hypokalemia (low potassium) because of unseemly emission of adrenocorticotropic hormone, as well as hyponatremia (low sodium) because of overproduction of antidiuretic chemical or trial natriuretic peptide.

Around one in three individuals with lung cancer foster nail clubbing, while 1 of every ten experience hypertrophic pneumonic osteoarthropathy (nail clubbing, joint touchiness, and skin thickening). Different immune system problems can emerge as paraneoplastic conditions in those with lung, including Lambert-Eaton myasthenic disorder (which causes muscle weakness), tactile neuropathies, muscle irritation, cerebrum swelling, and immune system decay of cerebellum, limbic system, or brainstem. Dependent upon one out of twelve individuals with cellular breakdown in the lungs have paraneoplastic blood thickening, including transient venous thrombophlebitis, clumps in the heart, and dispersed intravascular coagulation (clusters all through the body). Paraneoplastic disorders including the skin and kidneys are uncommon, each happening in up to 1% of those with lung cancer.

CHAPTER 2

DIAGNOSIS

PS: This section is highly recommended for Medical professionals; also feel to skip this chapter if you're not one

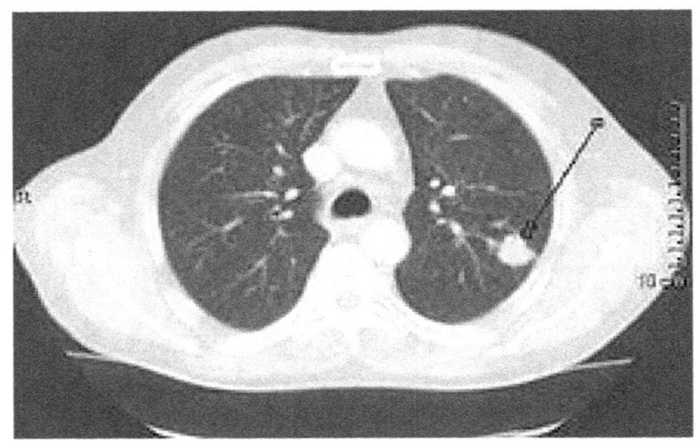

CT scan showing a cancerous tumor in the left lung

An individual suspected of having lung cancer will have imaging tests done to assess the presence, degree, and area of cancers. In the first place, numerous primary care providers perform a chest X-ray to search for a mass inside the lung. The X-ray might uncover an undeniable mass, the broadening of the mediastinum (suggestive of spread to lymph nodes there), atelectasis (lung breakdown), solidification (pneumonia), or pleural effusion; nonetheless, some lung growths are not noticeable by X-ray. Next, many go through computed tomography (CT) examining, which can uncover or reveal the sizes and areas of tumors.

A conclusive diagnosis of lung cancer requires a biopsy of the suspected tissue to be histologically analyzed for malignant growth cells (cancer cells). Given the area of lung tumors, biopsies can frequently be obtained by minimally invasive techniques: a fiber optic bronchoscope that can recover tissue (at times directed by endobronchial ultrasound), fine needle aspiration, or other imaging-directed biopsy through the skin. The people who can't go through a typical biopsy procedure may rather have a fluid or liquid biopsy taken (that is, a sample of some body liquid) which might contain circulating growth DNA that can be detected.

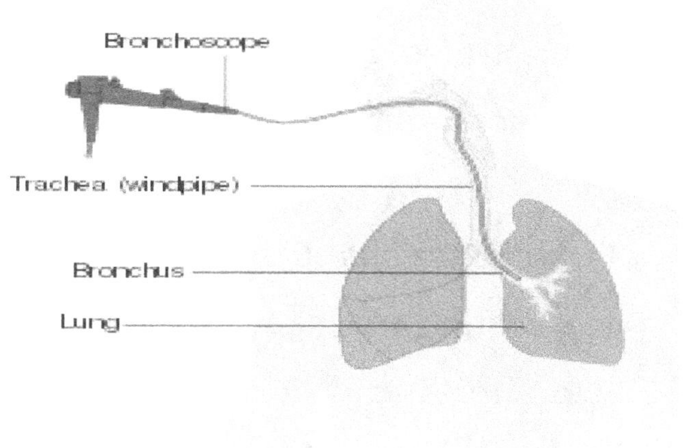

Diagram showing a bronchoscopy

Imaging is likewise used to examine the degree of cancer spread. Positron Emission tomography (PET) scanning or combined PET-CT scanning is frequently used to find metastases in the body. Since PET scanning is less delicate in the brain, the National Comprehensive Cancer Network suggests magnetic resonance imaging (X-ray) - or CT where X-ray is inaccessible - to scan the cerebrum for metastases in those with NSCLC and huge growths, or growths that have spread to the close by lymph nodes. While imaging recommends the growth has spread, the suspected metastasis is usually biopsied to affirm that it is cancerous. Lung cancer most usually metastasizes to the bones, liver, brain, and adrenal glands.

Cancer of the lungs can frequently show up as a solitary pneumonic nodule on a chest radiograph or CT filter. (A lung nodule or pulmonary nodule is a relatively small focal density in the lung. On the other hand, a solitary pulmonary nodule (SPN) or coin lesion, is a mass located in the lung a little smaller than 3 centimeters in diameter. A pulmonary micronodule has a diameter of say less than 3 millimeters)

In lung cancer screening, examinations as many as 30% of those screened have a lung nodule, most of which end up being benign. Other than lung cancer, numerous different illnesses can likewise give this appearance, including hamartomas, and granulomas brought about by tuberculosis, histoplasmosis, or coccidioidomycosis.

CLASSIFICATION

At diagnosis, lung cancer is classified in view of the types of cells the cancer is gotten from; tumors gotten from various cells progress and respond to treatment in a different way. There are two primary types of lung cancer, categorized by the size and appearance of the malignant cells seen by a histopathologic under a magnifying lens: small cell lung cancer (SCLC; 15% of cases) and non-small cell lung cancer (NSCLC; about 85% of cases).

SCLC cancers are much of the time found close to the center of the lungs, in the major airways. Their cells show up small with poorly defined boundaries, not much cytoplasm, many mitochondria, and have very distinctive nuclei with granular-like chromatin and no visible nucleoli.

NSCLCs contain a group of cancer types: adenocarcinoma, squamous-cell carcinoma, and large cell carcinoma. Almost 40% lung cancers are usually adenocarcinomas. Their cells grow in three-layered clumps, look like glandular cells, and may develop mucin. Around 30% of lung cancers are squamous-cell carcinomas. They regularly occur around large airways. The growths comprise sheets of cells, with layers of keratin. An empty or hollow cavity and related cell death are usually found at the focal point (center) of the tumor. Under 10% of lung cancers are large cell carcinomas, so named on the grounds that the cells are large, with overabundant cytoplasm, conspicuous nucleoli, and large nuclei. Around 10% of lung cancers are very rare types. These include blends of the above subtypes like adenosquamous carcinoma, and uncommon subtypes like carcinoid cancers, and sarcomatoid carcinomas.

A few lung cancer types are sub-classified in view of the development qualities of the cancer cells. Adenocarcinomas are classified as Lepidic (growing along the outer layer of intact alveolar walls), acinar and papillary, or micro papillary and solid pattern. Lepidic adenocarcinomas will quite often be least aggressive, while micro papillary and solid pattern adenocarcinomas are most aggressive.

Adding to cell morphology examination, biopsies are frequently stained by immunohistochemistry to confirm the classification of lung cancer. SCLCs bear the markers of neuroendocrine cells, for example, chromogranin, synaptophysin, and CD56. Adenocarcinomas usually express Napsin-A and TTF-1; squamous cell carcinomas need Napsin-A and TTF-1, however express p63 and its cancer-specific isoform p40. CK7 and CK20 are likewise normally used to separate or differentiate lung cancers. CK20 is usually found in several other cancers, however, missing in lung cancer. CK7 is present in lung cancers, however missing from squamous cell carcinomas.

SCREENING

Certain countries suggest that individuals who are at a high risk of developing lung cancer be screened at various intervals using low-dose CT lung scans. Screening programs might bring about early discovery of lung growths in individuals who are not yet experiencing symptoms of lung cancer, usually, early enough that the cancers can be treated successfully and result in decreasing mortality rate. There is proof that standard low-portion CT scans in individuals at high risk of developing lung cancer regulates and reduces the total lung cancer mortality rate by as much as 20%. In spite of proof of advantage in these populations, possible and potential harms of screening include the possibility for an individual to have a 'false positive' screening result that might prompt other unnecessary testing, distress, and invasive procedures. Even though uncommon, there is likewise a risk of radiation-induced cancer.

The US Preventive Service Task Force suggests yearly screening by using low-dose CT in individuals somewhere in the range of 55-80 who have a smoking history of say not less than 30 pack-years.

The European Commission likewise suggests that cancer screening programs across the European Union be stretched out in order to include low-dose CT lung scans for current or past smokers. Similarly, The Canadian Task Force for Preventive Health suggests that individuals who are current or previous smokers (with smoking history of more than 30 pack years) and who are between the ages of 55-74 years be evaluated for lung cancer.

PROGNOSIS

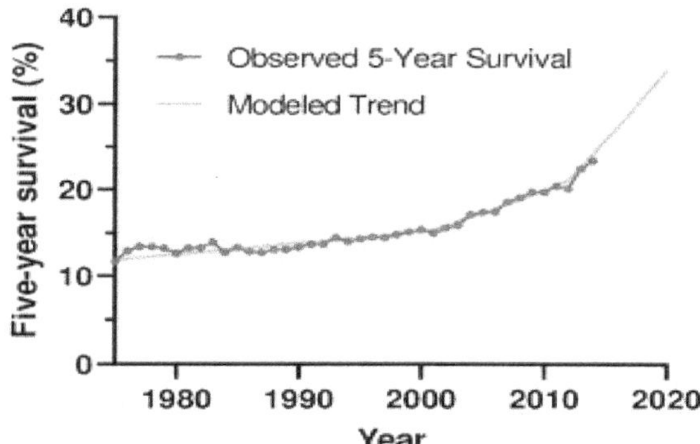

Percentage of individuals who survive 5 years from a lung cancer diagnosis over time, as per the NIH SEER program

About 19% of individuals diagnosed with lung cancer usually survive 5 years from diagnosis, even though prognosis differs in light of the phase and stage of the diseases at diagnosis and the type of lung cancer. Prognosis is better for individuals with lung cancer diagnosed at an early stage; those diagnosed at the earliest TNM stage, IA1 (little tumor, no spread), have a 2 year survival rate of 97% and five-year survival rate of 92%.

Those diagnosed at the most-advanced stage, IVB, have a 2 year survival rate of 10% and a five-year survival rate of 0%. Five-year survival rate is higher in ladies (22%) than men (16%). Women usually tend to be diagnosed with less-high level disease, and have better results or outcomes than men diagnosed at the very same stage. Average 5 years survival rate likewise varies across the world, with especially high 5-years survival rate in Japan (33%), and 5-years rate above 20% in 12 different countries:

Mauritius, Sweden, Canada, the US, South Korea, Taiwan, Israel, China, Latvia, Iceland, Austria, and Switzerland.

SCLC is usually aggressive. 10-15% of individuals survive 5 years after a SCLC diagnosis. Similarly as with other different type's lung cancer, the degree of sickness at diagnosis likewise affects prognosis. The average individual diagnosed to have limited stage SCLC survives 12-20 months from diagnosis; with broad stage SCLC around 12 months. While

SCLC usually responds at first to treatment, the vast majority at last relapse with chemotherapy-resistant cancer, getting through an average 3-4 months from the time of relapse. Those with limited stage SCLC that go into complete remission after chemotherapy and radiotherapy have a 50% chance of brain metastases developing in 2 years - a chance decreased by prophylactic cranial.

A few other individual and infection factors are related with improved and developed results. Those diagnosed at a more youthful age will generally have better results. The individuals who smoke or experience weight loss as a symptom will quite often have more regrettable and worse results. Cancer mutations in KRAS are related to reduced survival.

EXPERIENCE

The vulnerability and uncertainty of lung cancer prognosis frequently causes pressure, and makes future planning really troublesome and difficult, for those with lung cancer and their families. Those whose cancer goes into abatement often experience fear of their cancer reoccurring or advancing, related with low quality of life, negative mood, and functional disability. This dread is exacerbated by incessant or delayed reconnaissance imaging, and

*different   other   reminders   of
cancer risks.*

CHAPTER 3
CAUSES OF LUNG CANCER

Cancer of the lungs is caused by genetic damage to the DNA of lung cells. These changes are at times random, yet are regularly induced by taking in poisonous and toxic substances, for example, cigarette smoke. Cancer causing genetic mutations influence the cell's normal capabilities, including cell proliferation, modified cell death (apoptosis), and DNA repair. Ultimately, cells gain an adequate number of genetic changes to develop wildly, forming and developing a cancer, and at last spreading inside and beyond the lung. Uncontrolled cancer growth and spread causes the signs and symptoms of lung cancer. If unstopped, the spreading tumor will ultimately cause the demise of the affected person.

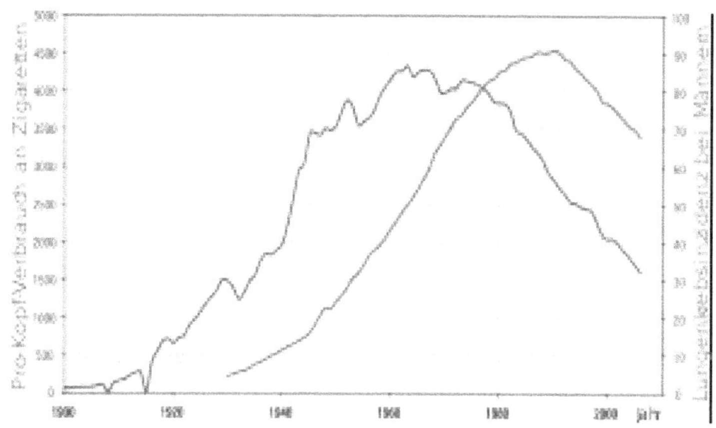

Relationship between cigarette consumption per person (in blue) and male lung cancer rates (dark yellow) in the United States

SMOKING

Tobacco smoking is a major contributor to lung cancer by

far, causing 80% to 90% of cases. With a high amount of cigarettes consumed, the risk of lung cancer also increases. Carcinogenic effects from tobacco smoking is because of different chemicals in tobacco smoke that cause DNA mutations, increasing the chance and risk of cells becoming cancerous. The International Agency for Research on Cancer identified not less than 50 chemical compounds in tobacco smoke as cancer-causing, and the most powerful is tobacco-specific nitrosamines. Exposure to these chemical compounds causes several kinds of DNA harm: DNA adducts, oxidative pressure, and breaks in the DNA strands.

Being around tobacco smoke - called passive smoking - can likewise cause cellular breakdown in the lungs (lung cancer). Living with a tobacco smoker increases one's risk of developing lung cancer by about 24%. An estimated stats proved that 17% of lung cancer cases in the people who don't smoke are caused by elevated degrees of environmental tobacco smoke.

Vaping might be a risk factor for lung cancer, yet in less proportion than that of cigarettes, and further research around the year 2021 is fundamental because of the time span it can take for lung cancer to develop after exposure to carcinogens.

The smoking of non-tobacco products isn't known to be

related with lung cancer advancement. Cannabis or marijuana smoking doesn't appear to independently cause lung cancer in the lungs - regardless of the high degrees of tar and known cancer-causing agents in marijuana smoke.

ENVIRONMENTAL EXPOSURE

Exposure to various other harmful chemicals - commonly experienced in certain occupations - is related with an increased risk of lung cancer. Occupational exposure to cancer-causing agents causes 9-15% of lung cancer. A good example is asbestos, which causes lung cancer by flaming the lung whether directly or indirectly. Exposure to all economically and commercial accessible types of asbestos increases the risk of cancer, and cancer risk increases with time of exposure.

Asbestos and cigarette smoking increases risk synergistically. That is; the risk of somebody who smokes and likewise has asbestos exposure dying is a lot higher than expected. Also, exposure to radon, a natural breakdown result of the earth's radioactive elements, is related to increased lung cancer risk. Radon levels vary with geography.

Underground miners have the best exposure; but even the lower levels of radon that seep into private or residential spaces can increase inhabitants' and occupants' risk of lung cancer. Like asbestos, cigarette smoking and radon exposure increases risk synergistically. Radon openness is responsible for 3% to 14% of lung cancer cases.

A few different chemicals experienced in different other occupations are likewise linked with increasing the risk of lung cancer including:

A. Arsenic used for the preservation of woods, pesticide application, and some ore smelting;

- ☐ *Ionizing radiation found during uranium mining;*
- ☐ *Vinyl chloride in papermaking;*
- ☐ *Beryllium in goldsmiths,*
- ☐ *Ceramic workers,*
- ☐ *Atomic or nuclear reactor workers, and*
- ☐ *Missile technicians;*

B. *Chromium in hardened steel creation, welding, and conceal tanning;*
- ☐ *Metal workers*
- ☐ *Nickel in electroplaters,*
- ☐ *Glass laborers,*

☐ *Welders, and*

☐ *Manufacturers of batteries, ceramics, jewelry, and diesel fumes found by miners.*

Exposure to air contamination, particularly particulate matter released by motor vehicle fumes and petroleum, increases the risk of lung cancer. Indoor air contamination from burning wood, charcoal, or crop residue for cooking and warming has likewise been connected to a high risk of developing lung cancer. The International

Agency for Research on Cancer has characterized emission from domestic burning of coal and biomass as carcinogenic.

OTHER DISEASE

Several other infections that cause inflammation of the lung increases one's risk of lung cancer. This connection is strongest for chronic obstructive pneumonic disorder- the risk is high in those with the most inflammation, and lower in those whose inflammation is treated with inhaled corticosteroids. Other inflammation lung and immune system illnesses, for example, tuberculosis, alpha-1 antitrypsin deficiency, scleroderma, interstitial fibrosis, Chlamydia pneumoniae infection, and HIV disease are related with high risk of developing lung cancer.

Epstein-Barr infection is related with the development of the rare lung cancer lymphoepithelioma-like carcinoma in individuals from

Asia, however not in individuals from Western nations. A role for a few other infectious agents- in particular human papillomaviruses, BK infection, SV40, JC infection, human cytomegalovirus, and measles infection, - in lung cancer development has been examined yet remains inconclusive as of 2024.

GENETICS

Specific gene combinations may make some individuals more helpless say susceptible to lung cancer. Close relatives of those with lung cancer have about twice the risk of developing lung cancer, even after controlling occupational and smoking habits. During my research, I was able to identify numerous gene variations related with lung risk, every one of which contributes a little risk increase. A large number of these genes contribute to pathways known to be engaged with carcinogenesis, named

DNA repair, inflammation, the cell division cycle, cell stress reactions, and chromatin remodeling. A few uncommon hereditary and genetic disorders that increases the risk of cancer and additionally increases the risk of lung cancer, named retinoblastoma and Li-Fraumeni syndrome.

CHAPTER 4
LUNG CANCER
PREVENTION

SMOKING SUSPENSION

The people who smoke can decrease their risk of lung cancer by stopping smoking - the longer one stays without smoking the greater the risk reduction is. Self-help programs have a little effect on progress of suspending smoking, though combined counseling and pharmacotherapy further improves discontinuance and smoking rates. The US FDA has supported and approved antidepressant treatments and the nicotine substitution varenicline as first-line treatments to aid smoking suspension. Clonidine and nortriptyline are suggested second-line therapies. Most of those diagnosed to have lung cancer try to stop smoking and about half succeed. Even after lung cancer diagnosis, smoking suspension further improves treatment results, lessening cancer treatment toxicity and disappointment and failure rates, and extending survival time.

At a societal level, smoking suspension can be enhanced by tobacco control policies that make tobacco items harder to get or use. Many of such policies are suggested or recommended by the WHO System Convention on Tobacco Control, endorsed by 182 nations, addressing more than 90% of the world's population. The WHO categorize these policies into 6 mediation categories, every one of which has been demonstrated and effective in lessening the cost of tobacco-induced disease burden on a population:

> i. *Increasing the cost of tobacco by increasing government taxes*
> ii. *Restricting tobacco use in broad daylight and public places to lessen exposure*
> iii. *Restricting tobacco advertising*

iv.   Publicizing the risks and harmful effects of tobacco products

v.   Approving help programs for those endearing to stop smoking and

vi.   Checking population-level tobacco use and the viability or effectiveness of tobacco control policies.

The more policies implemented, the higher the reduction. Lessening access to tobacco for young people is especially effective at reducing take-up of addictive smoking, and juvenile interest for tobacco products is especially delicate to increase in cost.

DIET AND LIFESTYLE

A few foods and dietary supplements have been related with lung cancer risk. High consumption of a few animal products - such as red meat (but not other meats or fish), saturated fats, as well as nitrosamines and nitrites (found in salted and smoked meats) - is related with a high risk of developing cancer of the lungs. Conversely, high consumption of vegetables and fruits is related with a lowered risk of lung cancer, especially cruciferous vegetables and fruits.

In view of the valuable and beneficial effects of vegetable and fruit supplementation of a few individual vitamins have been examined. Supplements with vitamin A or beta-carotene have no effect whatsoever on lung cancer, and on the other hand, heightens mortality rate. Dietary supplementation that contains vitamin E or retinoid comparably had no effect. Consumption of polyunsaturated fats, tea, beverages, coffee, and alcohol are completely connected with decreased risk of developing lung cancer.

Alongside diet, body weight and exercise as a habit are likewise connected with lung cancer risk. Being overweight is related with a lower risk of developing cancer, perhaps because of the propensity of the people who smoke cigarettes to have a lower body weight. But, being underweight is likewise connected with a lower lung cancer risk. I was able to prove in a few examinations that the individuals who work-out consistently or have healthier cardiovascular systems have a lower risk of developing lung cancer.

CHAPTER 5
TREATMENT OPTIONS

The treatment for lung cancer is overseen and managed by a group of experts from various departments who work together to give the most possible treatment.

This group includes the health specialist required to make a diagnosis, to stage your cancer and to design the best possible treatment.

The type of treatment you receive for the cancer of the lung depends upon a few variables, including:

- ☐ *The type of lung cancer you have (Small-cell or non-small cell mutation on the cancer)*
- ☐ *The size and position of the cancer*
- ☐ *How advanced is (the stage)*
- ☐ *Your general and overall health*

So deciding what treatment is best for you can be troublesome. Your cancer group/team will make suggestions, yet the final decision is your choice.

The most well-known treatment plans include a surgical process, radiotherapy, chemotherapy and immunotherapy. You may receive a combination of these treatments depending on the type and stage of your cancer.

YOUR TREATMENT PLAN

Your recommended therapy and treatment plan relies upon whether you have non-small cell lung cancer or small cell lung cancer.

A. Non-small cell lung cancer;

Assuming you have non-small cell lung cancer that is in just 1 of your lungs and you're doing well in your general health, you'll most likely have a medical surgery to remove the carcinogenic cells. This might be immediately followed by a course of chemotherapy to obliterate any carcinogenic cells that might have stayed in your body.

On the off chance that the cancer has not spread far however medical surgery isn't (for instance, because of your overall health means you have an increased risk of complications), you might be offered radiotherapy to obliterate the carcinogenic cells. At times, this might be joined with chemotherapy (also known as chemo radiotherapy).

In the event that the disease has spread excessively far for medical surgery or radiotherapy to be effective, chemotherapy and/or immunotherapy is usually suggested. And assuming the cancer begins to develop again after you have had chemotherapy treatment, one more course of treatment might be suggested.

At times, in the event that the cancer has a particular mutation, targeted or biological treatment might be suggested rather than chemotherapy, or after chemotherapy.

Biological treatments are meds that control or stop the development of cancer cells.

B. Small cell lung cancer;

*Small cell lung cancer is
normally treated with
chemotherapy, either all alone
or in mix with radiotherapy or
immunotherapy. This can assist
with prolonging one's life and
relieving all symptoms.*

*Surgery isn't typically used to
treat this sort of lung cancer.
This is on the grounds that the
cancer has currently spread to
different regions of the body by
its diagnosis.*

Nonetheless, assuming the cancer is seen very early, medical surgery might be used. In these cases, chemotherapy or radiotherapy might be given after a surgical process to assist with decreasing the risk of recurrence.

SURGERY

There are 3 primary types of medical procedure of lung cancer:

i. *Lobectomy - where 1 of the largest part of the lung (lobes) is taken out. Your specialists and doctors will propose this in the event that the cancer is in one part of the lung.*

ii. *Pneumonectomy - where the whole lung is taken out. This is used only when the cancer is situated in the lung or has spread all through the lung.*

iii. Segmentectomy - where a little piece of the lung is taken out. This system is just suitable for a few patients. It is possibly used assuming your doc thinks your cancer is little and restricted to one region of the lung. This is typically very early phase non-small cell lung cancer.

You might be worried about being able to breathe well if some or all your lungs are taken out, however it's very possible to inhale and breathe normally with just one lung. However, on the off chance that you have breathing issues prior to the operation, it's logical that these symptoms will go on even after surgery.

TESTS BEFORE MEDICAL

Before medical surgery, you'll need to conduct a few tests to check your general condition of

health and your lung function.
These can include:

An electrocardiogram (ECG) -
electrodes are used to screen
the electrical actions or activity
of your heart

A lung capability and function
test usually called spirometry -
where you'll inhale into a
machine which estimates and
measures how much air your
lungs can take in and out.
Lastly,

An exercise test

HOW IT'S PERFORMED

Medical surgery for the most part includes making a cut in your chest or side and taking out a segment or the entirety of the affected lung. This is known as a thoracotomy.

Close-by lymph nodes may likewise be taken out assuming it is presumed that the disease might have spread to them also.

Video-assisted thoracoscopic surgery (VATS), an alternative approach, may some of the time be appropriate. This is a type of keyhole medical surgery where little cuts are made in your chest. A little camera is embedded into one of the cuts, so the specialist can see the inside of your chest on a screen as they eliminate the part of the impacted lung.

AFTER THE SURGERY

You'll likely have the option to return home 5 to 10 days after your surgery. On the other hand, it can take numerous weeks to recuperate completely from a lung surgery.

After surgery, you'll be urged or encouraged to begin moving as soon as possible. Regardless of whether you need to remain in bed, you'll have to continue to do regular leg movements to help your circulation and prevent blood clusters from developing. A physiotherapist will show you breathing exercises to assist with preventing other complications.

At the point when you return home, you'll have to exercise delicately to develop your strength and wellness. Strolling and swimming are great types of exercises that are appropriate for the vast majority after treatment for lung cancer. Also see to it that you converse with your care team about which kinds of exercise are appropriate for you.

COMPLICATIONS

As with all medical surgery, lung surgery also has a risk of complications.

These can usually be dealt with using medication or more medical surgery, which might mean you need to remain in the hospital much longer.

Confusions of lung medical surgery can include:

- *Excessive bleeding*

- *Inflammation or contamination of the lung (pneumonia)*

- *A blood coagulation in the leg (vein thrombosis), which might actually travel up to the lung (pneumonic/pulmonary embolism)*

RADIOTHERAPY

Radiotherapy uses a pulse of radiation to annihilate cancer cells. There are various ways of treating lung cancer using this.

An intensive course of radiotherapy, known as radical radiotherapy, might be used to treat non-small cell lung cancer if by any chance you are not healthy enough for medical surgery. For tiny tumors, a unique kind of radiotherapy and stereotactic radiotherapy might be used rather than a medical procedure.

Radiotherapy can likewise be used to control the signs and symptoms, like pain and coughing up blood, and to lower the spread of cancer when a cure may not be possible (this is also known as palliative radiotherapy).

A sort of radiotherapy known as prophylactic cranial light (PCI) is in some cases used during the treatment of small cell lung cancer. PCI includes treating the entire cerebrum with a low portion of radiation. It's used as a preventive measure since there's a risk that small cell lung cancer will spread to your brain.

HOW RADIOTHERAPY IS GIVEN

The 3 fundamental ways that radiotherapy can be given are:

i. *Ordinary external beam radiotherapy - beams of radiation are directed at the affected parts of your body.*

ii. *Stereotactic radiotherapy - a more precise kind of external beam radiotherapy where a few high-energy beams convey a higher portion of radiation to the growth/tumor, while keeping away from the surrounding healthy tissue in every possible way.*

iii. *Internal radiotherapy - a slim tube (catheter) is embedded into your lung. A little piece of radioactive material is passed along the catheter and set against the growth for a couple of minutes, then moved.*

For lung cancer, external beam radiotherapy is used more frequently than internal radiotherapy, especially if it's presumed that cure is a possibility.

Stereotactic radiotherapy might be used to treat tumors that are tiny, as it's more viable and effective than standard radiotherapy alone in these conditions.

Internal radiotherapy is normally used as a palliative treatment when the cancer is hindering or partly impeding your airway.

COURSES OF TREATMENT

Radiotherapy treatment can be arranged in more ways than one.

Individuals having regular or conventional radical radiotherapy are probably going to have 20 to 32 treatment sessions. Radical radiotherapy is normally given 5 days per week, with a break at the end of the week (weekends). Every session of radiotherapy is 10 to 15 minutes and the course as a rule lasts 4 to 7 weeks.

Persistent hyper fractionated accelerated radiotherapy (Diagram or diagram) is an alternative approach to giving radical radiotherapy.

Chart is given 3 times each day for 12 days straight.

Stereotactic radiotherapy requires less therapy and treatment sessions in light of the fact that a higher portion of radiation is given during every therapy and treatment. Individuals having stereotactic radiotherapy for the most part have 3 to 10 treatment sessions.

Palliative radiotherapy for the most part includes 1 to 5 sessions.

SIDE EFFECTS

Side effects of radiotherapy to the chest can be:

☐ *Difficulties swallowing (dysphagia)*

☐ *Tiredness, Weakness, and Fatigue*

☐ *Hair loss on your chest (if you had any)*

☐ *Soreness and redness of the skin, which resembles and feels like sunburn*

☐ *Persistent cough that may bring up blood-stained phlegm*

Many and most individuals who have radiotherapy

experience little side effects or no side effects at all. Yet, you might have a few side effects during and after treatment.

Talk with your doc or physician or medical attendant for additional info about side effects and how to oversee or manage them.

Likewise, get clinical guidance assuming you're worried about your side effects.

CHAPTER 6
CAREGIVERS GUIDE

Being a caregiver for somebody with advanced lung cancer has a challenging task to do. Your job can change at different times as your loved one goes through therapy or treatment, in the event that they go into remission, and assuming that the cancer gets chronic.

Since most people with cancer aren't in the clinic all the time, home care has become more significant and important at this stage. A relative, work partner, or a friend who fills in as a caregiver turns into an important part of their loved one's medical care group.

Simultaneously, it's critical to let the individual with lung cancer take the lead in voicing out their necessities and making certain decisions.

TRY NOT TO DO IT ALONE

Since lung cancer usually has not many symptoms in its initial phases, individuals usually aren't diagnosed until it's chronic or advanced. At the point when somebody has stage 3 or 4 lung cancer that implies the disease has spread past their lungs. Alongside symptoms like troubled breathing and coughing they might experience fatigue, exhaustion, and pain. They could lose weight, and have nausea because of treatments such as chemotherapy and radiation.

This implies your loved one could need help with a few parts of their life, including emotional support, medical care, and everyday assistance around the house.

To ensure their necessities and wants are covered and to try not to wear yourself out, gather together a team to help. Loved ones can give meals, get things done (few errands), or simply invest time with your loved one to give you an opportunity to re-energize. Set up a list or bookkeeping sheet, or use an application like SignUpGenius or Lotsa Helping Hands to accumulate and coordinate your caregiving support team.

However, do not forget that loved ones have their own busy lives. So don't feel regretful in the event that you really need to employ somebody to do certain tasks, such as to do home upkeep or cleaning, whenever the situation allows.

HOW TO HELP WITH MEDICAL CARE

Give your loved one a chance to take the lead in their care as much as possible. Talk with them about their objectives: What do they want to achieve? What possible side effects would they say they are alright with? Would they like to join a clinical trial, where they'll have experimental drugs and treatments?

Get to know the specialists, nurses, and others in the medical care team so you feel comfortable with seeking clarification on certain issues. Make it a point of duty to ask any question during the appointment, however urge your loved one to speak up. Allow them to do the most part of the talking. In the event that you need a one-on-one discussion with the specialist, make a different appointment.

You can likewise support your loved one by:

i. *Taking notes during appointments to assist them with remembering vital points focuses*

ii. *Monitoring and keeping track of medication schedules and medication*

iii. *Giving rides to and from specialist's visits*

iv. *Monitoring a record of symptoms*

v. *Monitoring and keeping track of instruction for treatments such as chemotherapy vi.   Asking medical staff to teach you how to run certain medical task they'll need after surgery subsequent to leaving a hospital, like offering assistance with catheters*

You'll likely need to assist with the monetary, financial and legal aspect of your loved one's health care. At the point when you run into questions, you can go to experts like:

a. Hospital and clinic staff, patient navigator

who guide patients and their families step by step through the medical care process

b. *Insurance case manager and social, who can assist with insurance and charging claims and legal matters such as identifying a health care proxy.*

To ensure your loved one gets the care they need, talking about an advanced directive is significant. That is a legal report or documents that explains their wishes and desires for medical care, including:

If and when they'd decide to quit receiving treatment

Under what conditions they do or don't have any desire to be revived

Where they'd like to get end-of-life care, if necessary - in hospice, at a clinic, or at home

HOW TO HELP AT HOME

Cancer and its treatment leave your loved one with less time to manage and deal with the tasks of day to day life. So an enormous part of what a caregiver does happens at home. Alongside assisting with household errands, childcare, individual care, and other everyday tasks, you'll likewise have to manage side-effects that come from cancer and its treatment.

Nausea and loss or lack of appetite frequently go along with chronic or advanced lung cancer. Urge your loved one to eat, however don't bother or pressure them. To help, you can:

- ☐ *Serve 6-8 snacks or little meals a day rather than 3 big ones.*
- ☐ *Serve their food cold or at room temperature in the event that the smell of food is unpleasant.*
- ☐ *Offer smoothies or milkshakes rather than strong food.*
- ☐ *Offer plastic table knives or forks in the*

event that metal flatware's tastes terrible.

□ *Make eating a social event - sit with them and eat a meal regardless of whether they want to eat.*

Your loved one's doctor can refer you to a pro dietitian with a good track record and has worked with people who have cancer. Health insurance might cover expenses.

TO ASSIST YOUR LOVED ONE DEAL WITH FATIGUE

Assist them with setting up a plan of activities for the day, so they can zero in their energy on the things that are important to them.

At the point when they need to rest, tell companions and friends that they're not up for guests and allow calls to go to voicemail.

Exercise eases exhaustion and fatigue from cancer treatment, so assuming their doc or physician supports, go for strolls with them or assist them with doing certain scope-of-motion exercises.

Ensure your loved one's PCP is aware of any side effects or symptoms they're having after those exercises if there are any at all.

Their PCP or others in their health care team can likewise refer you to home care services, which assist with individual and personal care, fundamental health care, and many more. A portion of these services might be covered by medical or health insurance.

STEP BY STEP INSTRUCTIONS ON HOW TO OFFER EMOTIONAL SUPPORT

Managing and dealing with advanced lung cancer can cause your loved one to feel worried, angry, restless, apprehensive, or miserable - or even all these things at once. Since it's connected to smoking, there's often a stigma linked with lung cancer. That might raise feelings of disgrace or guilt.

You can in a gentle way invite your loved one to discuss their sentiments, feelings, and concerns. In any case, don't attempt to force them to talk before they're prepared. Tune in without passing judgment on their sentiments. It's alright to bring up reckless contemplations and self-

defeating thoughts, yet don't tell them to "cheer up" or "think positively".

Urge and encourage them to join a lung cancer support group, assuming they're up for that. Assuming that they appear to be discouraged or restless, talk with their care group about how the situation is playing out and what they're going through. They can refer them to both mental health resources and social support.

As they're capable, assist them with staying engaged with activities they love and enjoy. Try not to zero in so much on providing care that you don't take some time to appreciate and enjoy moments with your loved one. Managing difficulties together can bring you closer and help you both feel more confident and hopeful.

TAKE CARE OF YOU

Providing care is physical and emotionally depleting. So to be a viable and effective caregiver, you really need to look out for your own health and well-being. Take some time off (everyday if possible) to do something you love and enjoy. Remain connected with your friends. Get some physical activity, as well as relax with yoga or meditation.

Consider getting support for yourself through support groups or individual counseling. The American Cancer Society has a data set of support groups and forums for caregivers and cancer victims.

Providing care can also affect your work life, bringing about missed hours and absences. Once in a while it turns into a full time job. In the event that you're employed full-time, you might be given for as long as 12 weeks off every year to allow you to really focus on a sick friend, parent, or kid through the Family and Medical Leave Act (FMLA). While not all organizations and companies offer FMLA leave, you might have the option to get unpaid time off.

CHAPTER 7
JESUS THE SOLUTION

There's a solution to lung cancer permanently: The way is Jesus Christ!

There's no illness or disease, be it terminal that God can't heal.

Regardless of what has held one down, Jesus said In Matthew 11:28 " Come to me, all ye that are troubled and are heavy laden, and I will give you rest. Put on my weight, and learn from me; for I'm lowly in heart: and you will find rest for your souls. For my weight is not heavy but light."

Giving less regard to the conditions and problems you are going through Jesus can help you if only you have faith in him.

However, to do that, you must receive Jesus into your life. If by any chance you are yet to receive Jesus Christ, pray this with me:

"Dear Jesus Christ, I acknowledge that I am a sinner. I acknowledge that you died on the cross of Calvary for my sins, iniquity, and transgressions and rose again for the justification of my life. From now henceforth, I

acknowledge you as my Lord and my personal savior. Also, I decree that the hold and power of Sin, death, hell, and Satan is broken over my life for I'm in Christ Jesus now. Amen!"

The most significant and most important miracle has occurred because you believe and have faith in him. Trust God with your healing and every other problem.

Below are few bible texts that could be helpful to you;

Jeremiah 33:6, 1 pet 2:24 Jeremiah 30:17, Isaiah 38:16-17, Isaiah 57:18-29, Isaiah 40:29, Exo 23:24-26, … .. Run to Jesus now!!!

However, if you need counseling or guidance, connect with me one on one for free through this mail - will394560@gmail.com